HOW TO
STAY
HEALTHY

HOW TO STAY HEALTHY

A HANDBOOK FOR LIVING WELL

Jing Carter-Lu

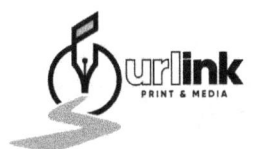

How to Stay Healthy

Copyright © 2024 by Jing Carter-Lu. All rights reserved.

No part of this publication may be reproduced, stored in a retrieval system or transmitted in any way by any means, electronic, mechanical, photocopy, recording or otherwise without the prior permission of the author except as provided by USA copyright law.

The opinions expressed by the author are not necessarily those of URLink Print and Media.

1603 Capitol Ave., Suite 310 Cheyenne, Wyoming USA 82001
1-888-980-6523 | admin@urlinkpublishing.com

URLink Print and Media is committed to excellence in the publishing industry.

Book design copyright © 2024 by URLink Print and Media. All rights reserved.

Published in the United States of America

Library of Congress Control Number: 2024920504
ISBN 978-1-68486-936-7 (Paperback)
ISBN 978-1-68486-939-8 (Digital)

23.09.24

Contents

Introduction 7
Chapter 1   Keep Your Home Clean 9
Chapter 2   Keep Indoor Air Cleaner..14
Chapter 3   Keep Your Body Clean and Healthy 19
Chapter 4   Keep Your Body's Immune System Strong............... 27
Chapter 5   Onion Treatment to Stop Fainting/Dizziness........... 28
Chapter 6   Food Medicines... 29
Chapter 7   Aromatherapy and Massage Therapy 35
Chapter 8   Daily Exercise 40
Chapter 9   Treat Dark Spots and Skin Tags 42
Chapter 10 Healing Dry Skin and Skin Maintenance................. 44
Chapter 11 Facial Massage for a Younger-Looking Face.............47
Chapter 12 Eczema Treatment 50
Chapter 13 Hair Loss Treatment 52
Chapter 14 Red Eye & Itchy Eye Treatment 54
Chapter 15 Hearing Health Maintenance 56
Chapter 16 Car Sickness Treatment...58
Chapter 17 Slam Your Fat Belly.. 60
Chapter 18 Body Cramp Treatment.. 65
Chapter 19 Treatment for Athlete's Foot 66
Chapter 20 Sauna Bath: Benefits and Caution..............................67
Chapter 21 Diabetes Care and Sugar Control in Meals................69
Chapter 22 Balance Body Energy for Mind Wellness 71
Chapter 23 Goal Setting for Your Career Success 75

Introduction

In 2020, people focused on fighting the COVID-19 disease and trying to stop it from spreading to more people. Sick people were isolated in hospitals for treatment. Facemasks were a must to go into stores and meetings, and six feet of social distance was required because the coronavirus was infectious and traveled through the air.

I was homeschooled in medicine since childhood because my father was a doctor and one of the managers who ran a medicine and medical equipment company. In 2020, I started testing many traditional food medicines and methods people used to stay healthy from cough and breathing problems to see if they could help us survive the COVID-19 pandemic. My test results were pretty good. I shared my writing with families and friends to help them survive the COVID-19 pandemic.

This book focuses on self-treatment and healthy maintenance to avoid getting sick from polluted air containing COVID-19, flu, etc. Food medicine can also improve the immune system, which your body pushes that virus out. Study the human body's acupressure points (also called acupuncture points), which really work to heal some pain symptoms and keep the body strong.

The best is that the methods listed in this booklet do not cost much, and you can do them yourself in the kitchen at home to stay healthy.

I also provide a solution and focus on addressing an important issue—indoor air quality. I introduce the Ceiling Vent Air Filter, Floor Vent Air Filter, and its holder product to help you clean your indoor air. Eco-safe Air Filter Manufacturing Company, based in the USA, makes these products. Filtering the air before it blows into each room in your house or apartment can help people stay healthier and avoid getting allergies from the dust.

We publish this booklet again with the new title "How To Stay Healthy", sincerely hoping that more people will benefit.

Chapter 1

Keep Your Home Clean

The routine household cleaning work we usually do involves:
- Vacuum the carpet area at least once per week
- Wipe down dust on all furniture once per week
- Mop the floor as needed and with a weekly cleaning schedule

If you have Pets in your home, I suggest you do these twice or thrice per week and do it as needed to keep your home clean.

During cleaning, open the Windows in the house to maintain a fresh air environment and ensure good ventilation.

MOLD CHALLENGE

Molds grow and spread like flower Pollen. It is floating in the air. We cannot see it with our naked eyes because they are so tiny/little and lightweight. You might see it under the microscope in the Research Laboratory. They grow wherever they land. We will see them when they grow bigger. At home, we see the mold returning to our bathtub's edge, the bottom part of the shower curtain, and the wall. That is why we must clean and brush the bathtub with bleach to remove the mold stains at least once weekly.

There are three things that we can do to clean it out:

(1) Brush it with liquid or powdered bleach cleaning products.

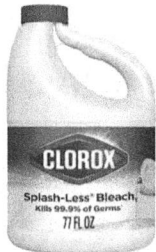 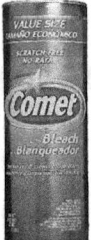

(2) Spray the Mold Remover on the black/ pink Mold spots to remove it.

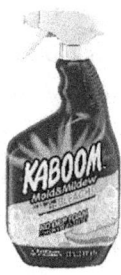

(3) Use a Ceiling Vent Air Filter to prevent Mold from circulating in your home, especially in the bathroom.

Patent Technology
US 9,352,259

ECO-SAFE AIR FILTER MANUFACTURING COMPANY

A Solution To Stop Mold Spores Circulate In the House

Healthier & Happier® *Ceiling/Floor* Vent's *Eco Air Filters*

Contact Info:
Tel: 1 (678) 900-6617
www.EcosafeAirFilters.com

To order, send email to:
sales@EcosafeAirFilters.com

Where are mold grow in family housing?

A: **It could be any where due to moisture.**
See pictures on the side. You've probably heard the old saying that an ounce of prevention is worth a pound of cure. That is certainly true when it comes to household mold. Mold in the home can <u>damage the home</u> itself and cause <u>serious health problems</u>. Mold remediation can cost thousands and thousands of dollars. Preventing mold in the first place is usually much easier and much more affordable. While you cannot always prevent mold, there are many things you can do to reduce the likelihood of a household mold problem from developing.
Ref.: www.mold-answers.com

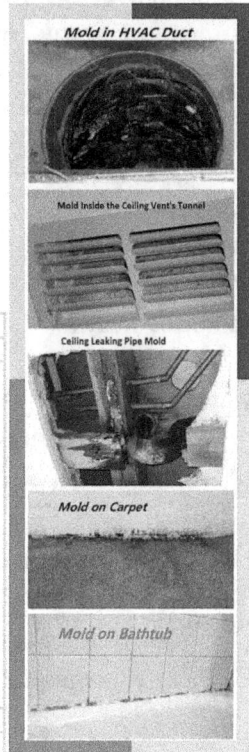

E co-safe Air Filter
　　　Manufacturing Company
◆ ◆ ◆ ◆ ◆ ◆ ◆ ◆ ◆

We provide customized sizes service.
No job is too small. Customer satisfy guaranteed.

About Us:
We identified the problem: Mold, Fungi, Dust Mites, and Insects may exist in the ceiling vents and air duct, particularly the bathroom's Ceiling Vent, due to moisture. The blow back of harmful mold spore airborne into rooms may cause occupants to suffer from allergies, headache, eczema, etc. ...
The solution to solve problem, is our innovation products - Ceiling/Floor Vent's Eco Air Filters.

Benefits of Product: Healthier & Happier® is our passion!
 1) STOP Indoor Air Pollution by filtering out mold spores.
 2) Prevent Bugs Coming into Rooms from Vents.
 3) Easy use: 2 sides filtration technology.
 4) Save Money: Washable & Reusable. Up to one year.
 5) No Waste: 100% Recyclable.

BUG CHALLENGE

We all have experienced spiders, ants, roaches, etc., entering our homes. We do not know how and where they enter; however, those bugs are in our environment.

What could we do to stop the bugs from coming into our homes?

a) Spray some of the Cockroach killer on the Kitchen floor's corners and under the sink area, where the bugs possibly hide.
b) In the closet or wherever you store clothes, use old-fashioned Moth Balls, which can kill Clothes Moths and their Eggs and Larvae.
c) Use "Ceiling Vent Air Filters" and "Floor Vent Air Filters" to prevent bugs and dust mites from entering through the A/C system's vents, which blow air into the rooms of the house.

REMOVE THE ODORS AT HOME

Sometimes, we smell something bad at home. We must find out what is causing the bad smell and get things cleaned out to maintain good family health.

Here are a few tips for removing odors at home:
a) To remove odors from the refrigerator, put an opened box of baking soda. This can also help keep food fresh for a longer time.
b) To remove the odor from shoes, put a few pieces of the old-fashioned mothballs into the shoe closet or shoeboxes. Sometimes, the odor is inside the shoes due to sports activities that cause people's feet to sweat in the shoes. The wet condition could make the shoes smell bad.
   Treatment: Use a hammer to mash a few pieces of the mothballs. Put some of the moth balls' powder inside each shoe. Then, put the shoes under sunlight during noontime for two to three hours. This will remove the odor completely from your shoes.
c) To remove odors in the microwave oven, put a half cup of vinegar into a microwaveable bowl and put the bowl into the microwave oven. Then, put the microwave on high for one minute to heat the vinegar. If necessary, add another minute on the high setting. You will notice the odors in the

microwave oven have disappeared. Plus, the microwave oven will become amazingly easy to clean. Use a warm, wet towel to wipe the inside of the microwave oven.

Here are a few tips for removing Odors on the human body:
a) To remove odors from your hair, put two to three spoonfuls of baking soda into a large pot of warm water and stir it slowly until it dissolves completely. Soak your hair into the mixture, gently rub the scalp, and comb through the hair for about ten minutes. Then, use shampoo to wash your hair as you usually do. Repeat it every two to three days until the hair odor is removed.
b) To remove the odor in your mouth, brush your teeth in the morning and before bedtime. Use a hydrogen peroxide topical solution (a first aid antiseptic oral debriding agent) or the refreshing mint mouthwash and gargle solution to gargle for two to three minutes right after brushing your teeth in the morning and before bedtime. It is important not to eat any food or candy after cleaning your mouth at bedtime.
c) Option 1: chewing a few pieces of roasted peanuts in the daytime when you smell bad breath.
    Option 2: chewing a Double-mint bubble gum can help keep the bad smell away from the mouth.
d) When a person reaches puberty, special hormones affect the glands in the armpits. These glands make sweat that can smell. Use armpit deodorant that has twenty-four-hour protection every day. And especially during the summertime, take a shower and roll a little deodorant onto your armpits as often as needed. If it's seriously affecting your social and family life, you can see a doctor for surgery, which will resolve the issue.

Chapter 2

Keep Indoor Air Cleaner

We sincerely introduce the innovative Ceiling Vent Air Filters and Floor Vent Air Filters that are newly available in the market. These Vent Air Filters are designed to help maintain a healthier indoor air environment. Their brand is HEALTHIER & HAPPIER®. The Ceiling Vent Air Filter products can significantly benefit those who use them. Here are some facts demonstrating the effectiveness of filtering out dust and the ease of use of the Ceiling Vent Air Filter Holder and its Air Filter Sheet:

Firstly, it is a simple product. The "Ceiling Vent Air Filter" package includes everything you need for a simple and quick installation process on the A/C vent where the air blows into your room. You can start using it right away without any hassle. You will experience the benefits of filtered cleaner air in the comfort of your home.

The "Ceiling Vent Air Filter" package includes a white plastic Ceiling Vent Air Filter Holder and its Air Filter Sheet 8" x 16" inches, and five pieces of Drywall Screws for easy installation. It is specially designed to cover various ceiling vent and well vent sizes, including 8"x16", 8"x14", 8"x12", 6"x14", 6"x12", 6"x10", 4"x14", etc.

The "Floor Vent Air Filter" package includes a white plastic Floor Vent Air Filter Holder and its Air Filter Sheet 4" x 12" inches, and four pieces of Drywall Screws for easy installation. It is specially designed to cover multiple floor and wall vents of various sizes, including 4"x12", 4"x10", 4"x8", 2"x10", etc.

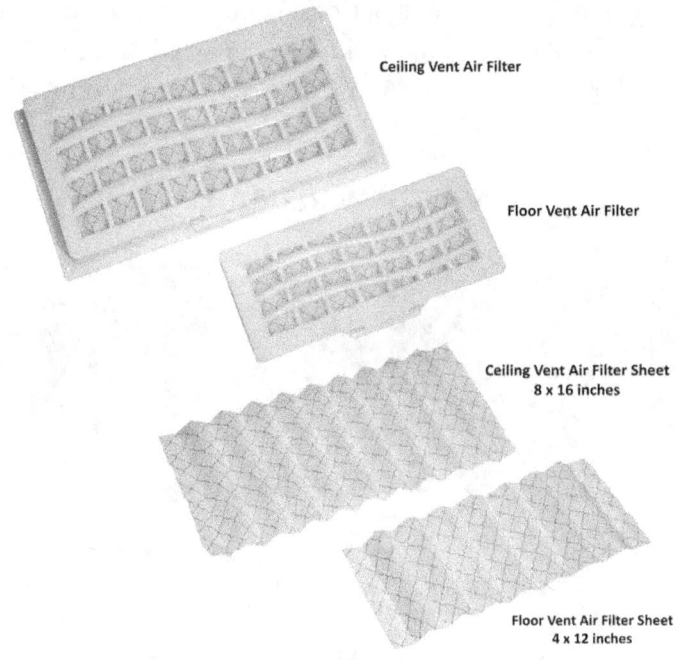

Secondly, it is easy to use. Open the cap on the holder and replace the Air Filter Sheet every six months.

HOW TO USE IT

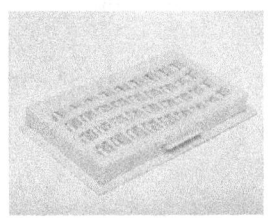

Ceiling Vent Air
Filter Holder

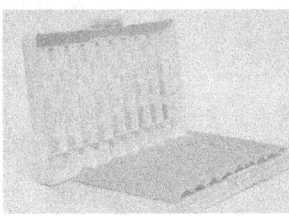

Open the cap
add Eco Air Filter
Sheet, Merv 8

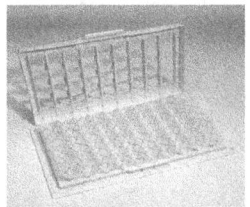

Open the cap
add Air Filter Sheet,
Merv 5

Thirdly, it efficiently filters out dust. Look at the air filter sheets after six months of use, and you will see how much dust they collected. You may be breathing in some dust without the Ceiling Vent Air Filter.

USAGES DEMONSTRATED

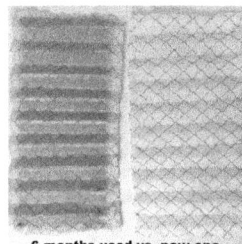 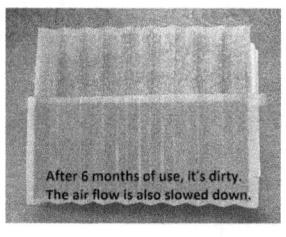 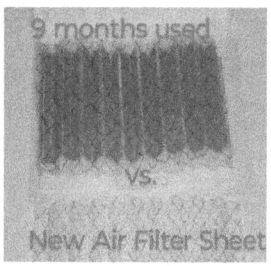

| Six months used | Six months used | Nine months used |
| Air Filter Sheet, Merv 5 | Eco Air Filter Sheet, Merv 8 | Air Filter Sheet, Merv 5 |

As you can imagine, dust will blow straight into your room if not filtered by the ceiling vent air filter. These unique products are created and manufactured by Eco-safe Air Filter Manufacturing Company in GA, U.S.A. If you have questions or inquiries, please send your request through email to sales@ EcosafeAirFilters.com

Finally, it is a must-have product for every home and school, especially for households with babies and seniors. Ceiling and Floor Vent Air filters can provide cleaner indoor air and reduce the risk of allergies and flu.

Below are some pictures that demonstrate how the Ceiling Vent Air Filters and Floor Vent Air Filters work:

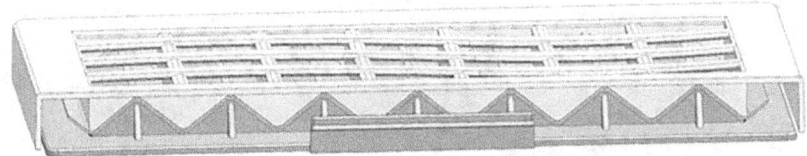

The pink color shows the AIR FILTER SHEET inside the Holder

A DISPLAY WHERE THE CEILING VENT AIR FILTERS WERE USED

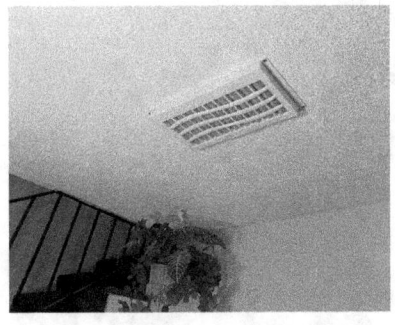
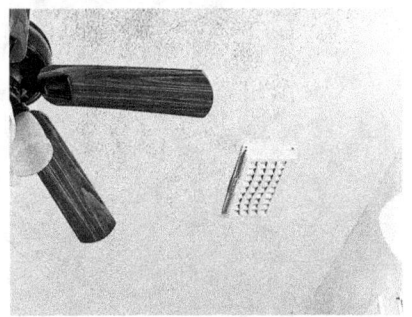

Used on the first floor AC ventUsed on the bedroom AC Vent

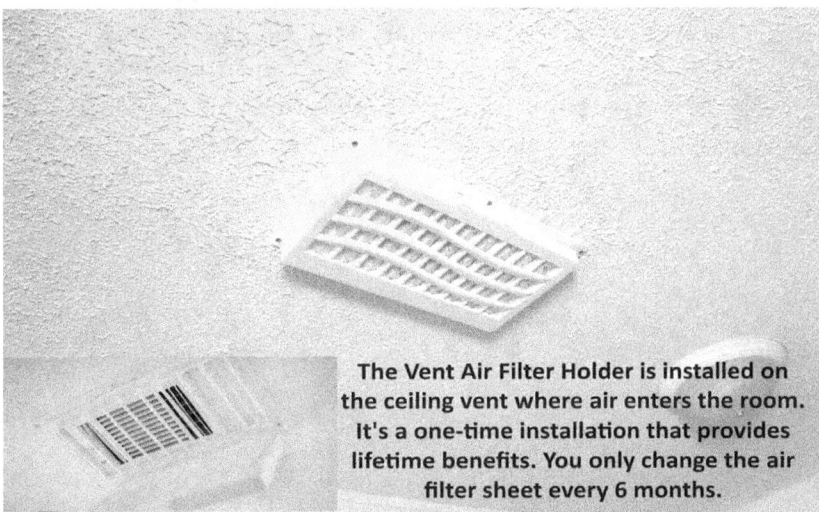

The Vent Air Filter Holder is installed on the ceiling vent where air enters the room. It's a one-time installation that provides lifetime benefits. You only change the air filter sheet every 6 months.

A Ceiling Vent Air Filter was installed on the AC vent in the kitchen.

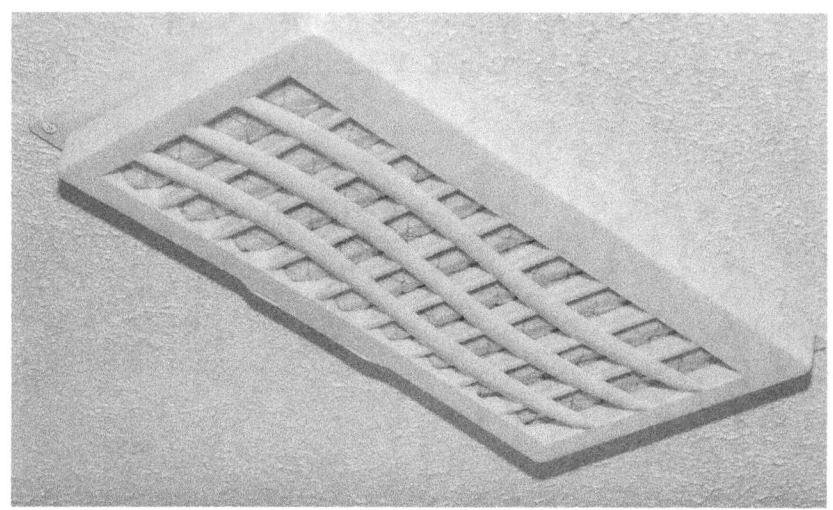

A Ceiling Vent Air Filter was installed on the AC vent in the living room.

We wish every family to achieve a healthier and safer indoor air environment.

Chapter 3

Keep Your Body Clean and Healthy

Medical research and studies show that our hands might contain some bacteria and germs when we work and touch something unclean. If we eat food with uncleaned hands, the chances are that we are taking some of the bacteria and germs into our stomachs.

I highly recommend you do the following to avoid getting sick often.
- a) Use soap to wash your hands before eating meals.
- b) Take a warm shower with soap each day.
- c) Drink a half cup of warm salt water (just a little salt) after you get up in the morning. It helps clean your stomach.
- d) Drink Green Tea in the morning during/after Breakfast.

DRINK CLEAN WATER DAILY

Water helps your body stay healthy. You can buy purified water bottles from stores or make clean water at home or in the office.

Boiling the water from the pipe to 100 °C for a few minutes will remove and purify all possible microorganisms. So the water becomes safe for people to drink.

Researchers studied the best water amount for children and adults, from 4 cups to 8 cups. Of course, you can adjust the amount based on your body's needs.

TREAT AN ITCHY AND/OR PAINFUL THROAT

If you feel an itch inside your throat and/or nostril and are sneezing, you must take care of yourself immediately. This happens when you breathe dusty or allergic air through your nose and mouth.

a) Use Sinus Wash Bottle and its Sinus Wash Refill packets to rinse it.

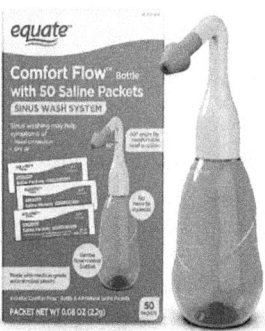

b) Hydrogen peroxide (first aid antiseptic oral debriding agent) can be used as an oral gargle and rinse agent. See the referenced product picture below.

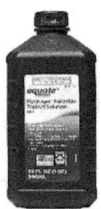 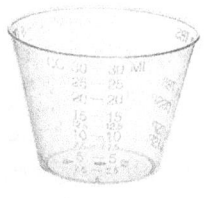

Use directions: Fill a cup with 15 mL of the solution, swish the undiluted solution in your mouth for one minute, then spit out the solution. Do this after breakfast and before bedtime while you have an itchy and painful throat or bleeding gums while brushing your teeth. Or use it as needed when you feel itchy or in pain.

TREAT ITCHY AND PAINFUL NOSTRILS

Use Hydrogen Peroxide (Topical Solution USP) as the **cleansing solution**

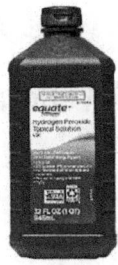 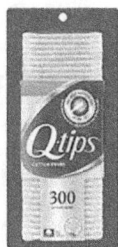

These are the directions for use: Put a small amount of the hydrogen peroxide into a small container, dip two cotton swabs into the solution to wet the cotton, and use the soaked cotton swabs to clean each nostril. You will see white things being cleaned out, which is normal. Clean it as often as necessary to stop the itch and pain in your nostrils.

Hydrogen peroxide acts as a first-aid antiseptic for treating minor cuts and abrasions.

Most of the time, we feel our throats itchy and painful because of cold. For example, when the weather changes from summer to fall, we haven't added more clothes yet, and the cold air blows on our bodies, making us feel cold.

THE QUICK RECOVERY METHOD FOR COLD

1. Make some ginger tea to drink while it's warm. Rest well in bed for a few hours to recover fast. You can stop the cold within one day when you treat it at the very beginning of the symptom. Otherwise, it takes a week to recover from cold symptoms, such as runny nose, cough, throat pain, headache, etc.

    Preparation: Cut the ginger (2–5 g) into small pieces. Boil it in the pot with a full bowl of water. When the water

is boiling, turn the stove to low heat to continue cooking the ginger for ten minutes. Add a half spoonful of dark-brown sugar right after you remove it from the stove. The ginger tea is ready. Drink it when it's warm.
2. Putting some warm clothes on when you go outdoors.

TREAT SKIN THAT'S ITCHY FROM BUG BITES

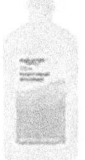

70 percent isopropyl alcohol

If you feel itchy, use 50–70 percent isopropyl alcohol (also called rubbing alcohol) to rub your skin where you were bitten by a mosquito or other tiny bug. It will help stop the itch.

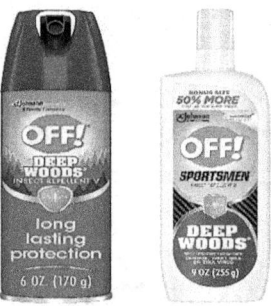

Deep Woods insect repellent

Use OFF! Deep Woods insect repellent to prevent bug bites. Spray some insect repellents on your body before going outdoors so you won't get bites.

Mosquito bites usually bump the bitten spot, making you scratch yourself until you break your skin. For persistent itching on the skin due to bug bites and scratch infections, use hydrogen peroxide (topical solution USP) as a cleansing solution for the affected area. It can help stop the itching and act as an antiseptic.

The hydrogen peroxide topical solution is a particularly important first aid antiseptic oral debriding agent for people in the southern part of the United States, such as South Carolina, Georgia, Alabama, Texas, Florida, etc. The hot and humid weather during the summer months creates a rich environment for bugs and bacteria to grow.

In the southern part of the United States, things in the air start appearing during the springtime. The wind blows pollen into the air, which can land everywhere—on streets, cars, roofs, etc. It can cause allergies in people's eyes, noses, skin, etc.

We also see some tiny spiders and other kinds of tiny bugs sized like a little dot or a period in writing. When those little bugs have been blown onto people's skin/clothes when we go under trees or closer to an area with trees, they could cause people's skin to itch. Those tiny spiders have colors like red, light yellow, semi-clear, white, and black. They can make people's skin itch and cause red dots to appear. Therefore, we must keep up with the cleaning maintenance to maintain a healthy body by showing up every day in Summer.

TREAT SUNBURNED SKIN

Use sunscreen lotion to prevent sunburn. I suggest the Waterproof Sunscreen Lotion Intensive UV Sunblock cream— SPF50 + Moisturizing Skin. During the summer, we sweat a lot. The waterproof sunscreen lotion could help us avoid sunburn for the whole day.

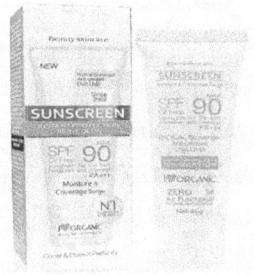

Waterproof Sunscreen Lotion

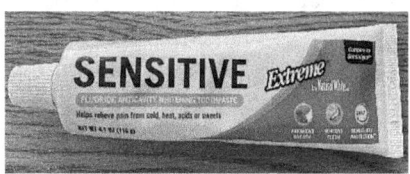

Sensitive Toothpaste

This special Sensitive Extreme toothpaste from Natural White can help relieve pain from cold, heat, acids, or sweets in the gums (medically called "gingiva"). We can also use the toothpaste for a small patch of itchy or painful skin from minor burns due to sunburns, hot water, or hot oil. It not only stops pain in the gums and skin due to minor cuts but can also stop the itchy feeling on the skin due to insect bites and sunburns.

TREAT ITCH OR PAIN IN THE ANUS

The anus (also called asshole) is the opening in a person's bottom through which solid waste leaves the body. It might get irritated by the waste from time to time each day, causing it to itch or feel painful.

You can keep it clean and treat the itch/pain when it occurs by using Epsom salt. You will need the following items in the pictures below:

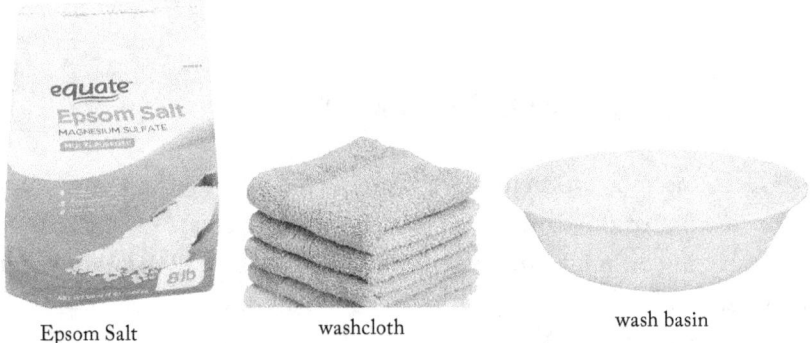

Epsom Salt   washcloth   wash basin

Epsom salt (magnesium sulfate) soaks minor sprains and bruises. Now we use Epsom salt to stop the anus itching.
    a) Grab a handful of Epsom salt and put it in the washbasin (the size should be large enough for you to soak your bottom in).
    b) Take a small washcloth and fill the washbasin one-third full of hot water to dissolve the Epsom salt.

c) When the temperature is warm enough to soak your hand in, soak your bottom in the warm/hot water for ten minutes in the washbasin.
d) Use the small washcloth to gently clean the itchy or painful place while it is soaked in the warm Epsom salt water.

Women occasionally get a vulva itchy; use a washcloth to clean the itchy spot while it is soaked in warm Epsom salt water until it stops feeling itchy. Remember to check the temperature of the Epsom salt water. It should be around 70–75 °C (Celsius) or 158–167 °F (Fahrenheit). According to research data, E. coli and most bacteria lose their activity when the temperature increases to 75 °C.

The temperature of boiling water is 100 °C, which can burn your hand, so a temperature of 70–75 °C would not burn your hand or butt. You will feel the warmth when you test the water with your hand, but you will not get burned by it.

TREATING PINWORMS

This type of worm is very tiny, is white, and has a little black needlelike tip on one of its ends. It is about 0.5–1 cm long and less than 0.1 cm thick, and the other end is its reproductive side; it moves this around, making you feel itchy. When people use fingers to scratch it, the worm's eggs and/or larvae will be attached to the skin on your fingers. If people use their fingers to eat food, the eggs and/or larvae will go back into their stomachs and become the adult worm, and this can cause the anus to feel itchy again. That is the life cycle of the pinworm.

People must wash their hands after using the bathroom to poop. Poop is also called excrement or shit. Poop is an incredibly good source of nutrition for plants. It is commonly used to grow vegetables, flowers, and trees.

There are two treatment methods for pinworms. To stop the pinworm from moving its tail around to cause the itchy anus, smooth a big chunk of petroleum jelly on the anus after washing and soaking it with the warm Epsom salt-water solution. Petroleum jelly can stop the worm from moving around and stop the itch.

Based on medical studies, these kinds of bug problems at the anus happen when we eat raw vegetables and when we eat food with our fingers without washing our hands.

To avoid getting the worm from food, we can steam the vegetables or cook vegetables with meat for meals.

Always wash fruit with warm salt water, then add a small spoonful of flour and soak in five minutes. Then, wash and rinse with cold water.

Once you've stopped the worms from coming into your body through the mouth and fingers, one or two weeks later, you wouldn't have the anus itch problem that was caused by the pinworm.

Treat the itchy spot as often as needed.

Chapter 4

Keep Your Body's Immune System Strong

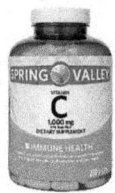 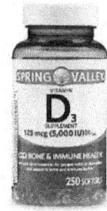 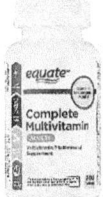

1. Take one piece of Complete Multivitamin per day.
2. Take one piece of Vitamin C daily to increase the immune system health.
3. Take one piece of Vitamin D3 daily to increase bone and immune health. I highly recommend you add a piece of Vitamin C and a piece of Vitamin D3 to your regular Complete Multivitamin to increase your immune system so that the Coronavirus has less chance to affect you and make you sick.
4. Chicken Soup: Make the chicken soup at home once weekly for your body and soul.
5. Eat more beans. Most Beans contain some Isoflavones, a combination of wrinkle-reducing isoflavones that help your body stay young.
6. Eat three meals per day regularly. Eat more at lunchtime and less during dinnertime.
7. Re-energize your body by taking 30- to 60-minute rest/or nap after Lunch.

Chapter 5

Onion Treatment to Stop Fainting/Dizziness

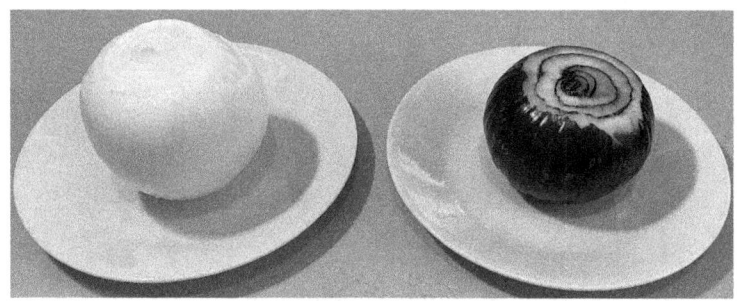

Yellow or Purple
It doesn't matter as long as they are Onions.

When you feel a little bit of short of breath, dizzy and a slight cough (any one of the symptoms), do the Onion Treatment.

Cut a fresh Onion (see pictures). We smell and breath in the Onion's smell odour from nose, take a deep breath down to the chest, then breath it out from mouth. Do it 20 times. It can stop the fainting for people.

Based on the herb study, the Onion's smell odour has a function to treat germs away that might possibly attach on the wall membrane inside of our breath system. Such as, inside the nostrils, throat, lung, etc.

After smelling it, put the Onion by bedside. The Onion can absorb some germs in the air away from you.

Chapter 6

Food Medicines

Food Medicine is useful for maintaining good health and treating symptoms initially for fast healing and recovery. If you have a serious medical situation that involves a severe combination of symptoms, I advise you to see a doctor.

3 METHODS THAT CAN STOP COUGHING

Coughing is the most common symptom people experience when they feel sick. Here I share the three most efficient food medicines for treating cough symptoms.

METHOD 1: ROCK SUGAR & PEAR JUICE

Materials include One pear and a few pieces of rock sugar.

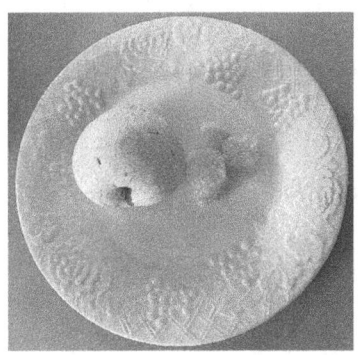
One Pear and pieces of rock sugar

→

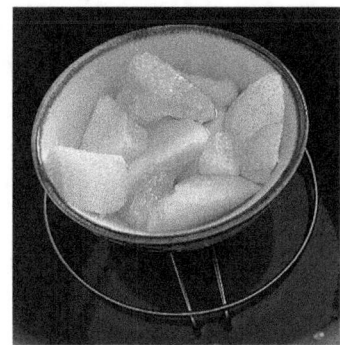
Prepare to steam in the pot

Cut the Pear into smaller pieces and remove the core. Steam the pear and a few pieces of rock sugar together in a bowl full of water (see pictures above) for fifteen minutes. Eat the Pear and drink the juice when it is warm. Eat this for three to five days as light refreshment and rest well. When you take deep breaths, you will feel your lungs getting clearer and better each day. You should be healed from the coughing sickness.

METHOD 2: GARLIC JUICE

Materials include seven cloves of Garlic and a few pieces of Rock Sugar.

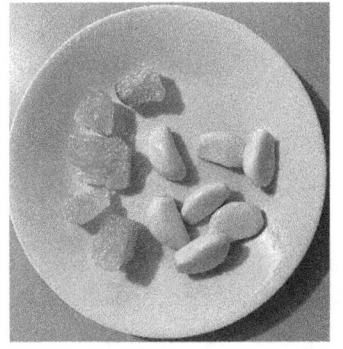
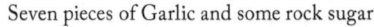
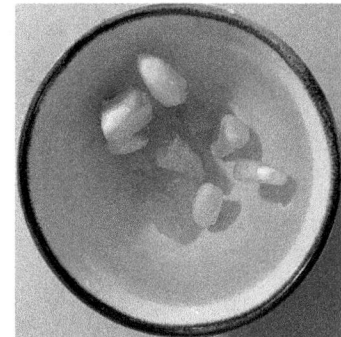

Seven pieces of Garlic and some rock sugar   Prepare to steam for fifteen minutes

You can also cut the garlic into small pieces if you don't like to bite into the whole piece. The juice from garlic is also a key element in food medicine. Steam the garlic and a few pieces of rock sugar in a bowl full of water together (see pictures above) for fifteen minutes. You will see the rock sugar melt into the Garlic Juice. Drink the juice when it is warm.

METHOD 3: EGGPLANT'S BASE JUICE

Materials include a few Eggplant base parts.

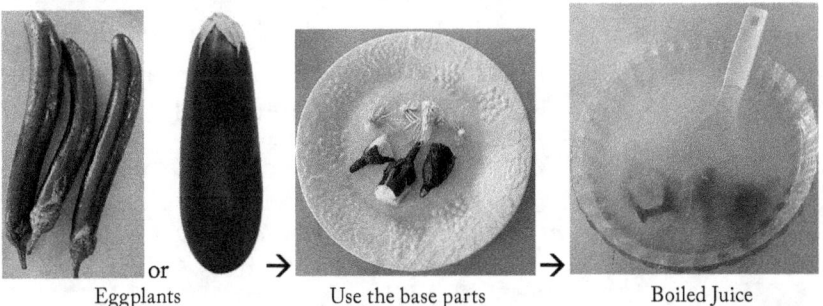

Eggplants → Use the base parts → Boiled Juice

Boil eggplants' base parts (roots from green onion are optional) with a full bowl of water (about 0.75 Liters) in the pot to boil for fifteen minutes. Drink the juice when it is warm. Do this in the morning. You can use it twice daily; boil it again in the afternoon and drink the juice. Use a fresh eggplant base part for the next day. Take this for a continued three to five days, and rest well. The cough will be stopped. Some people said it stopped their many years of chronic cough. Eggplant is an eatable vegetable and is safe for everybody in the family to try, including young children.

CLEAN YOUR BODY'S BLOOD CLOTS

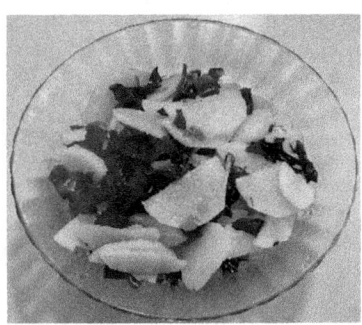

Wood Ear cooked with Common Yam

Materials include Wood Ear fungus. The Wood Ear fungus is an herbal medicine ingredient that has been recorded hundreds of years ago in the Chinese Herb Medicine Books.

Here, we emphasize the benefit of wood ears; they can reduce and clean the blood clots from the human body. You can add the wood ear to meat soup, cook it with egg, or cook it with vegetables. Eating Wood Ear keeps your body strong and healthy, which can help you stay safe from the COVID-19 pandemic.

Here are instructions for preparing the raw materials:

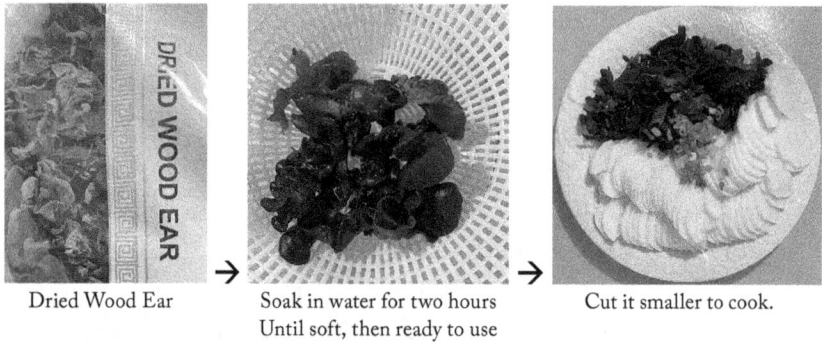

Dried Wood Ear → Soak in water for two hours Until soft, then ready to use → Cut it smaller to cook.

Grab a handful of dried wood ear (about 1 gram) and sock it in a bowl of warm water. After two hours, you will see it enlarged and become soft, as in the picture shown above.

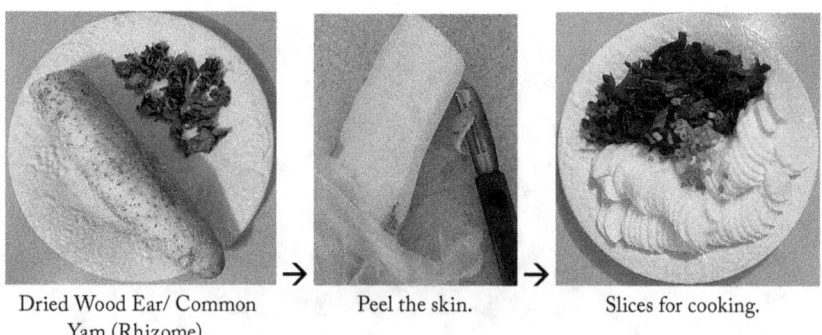

Dried Wood Ear/ Common Yam (Rhizome). → Peel the skin. → Slices for cooking.

When peeling the yam's skin, hold it in a plastic bag. Some of the points on the Yam's skin may make your hand itch.

The Common Yam (Rhizome) has the core function of promoting digestion and blood circulation. It can also lower blood sugar, benefit the lungs, and relieve cough. Additionally, it can aid in the prevention of cardiovascular and cerebrovascular diseases. Yam is rich in mucus protein, vitamins, and trace elements, which can well inhibit the deposition of blood lipids onto the vascular wall, playing the role of pro-longevity.

FOODS THAT MAKE THE IMMUNE SYSTEM STRONG

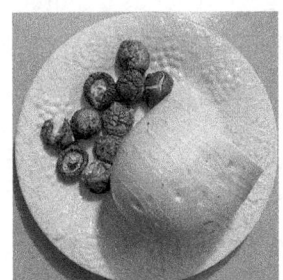
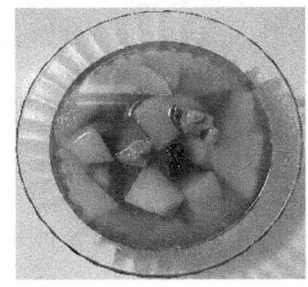

White Radish and Mushroom Soup

Here are instructions on how to prepare the White Radish and Dried Mushrooms:

Soak the dried mushrooms in warm water for two hours in a bowl. Cut them in the middle to check if they are ready to cook. They are ready for cooking when they become soft inside the root part.

Cut the white radish into the smaller pieces you like for your soup.

The following are the benefits of consuming white radish:

a) *Prevention of cancer.* The cellulose in white radish helps the body discharge metabolic waste and maintain a healthy state. In addition, the lignin in white radish can decompose ammonium nitrite in the blood. Ammonium nitrate is a harmful substance that causes cell cancellation. Edible white radish can help anybody eliminate cancer cells, thus preventing cancer.

b) *Cools the blood to prevent bleeding.* White radish is cooling; it can get rid of lung heat and treat oral ulcers caused by heat toxins in the body, sores in the mouth and tongue, a dry pharynx by having it sweat, and other symptoms. Many people get a headache or feel a heavy head because of overdrinking alcoholic products. White radish can help reduce the problem.

c) *Promote digestion.* The cellulose content in white radish is rich; it can promote gastrointestinal peristalsis, help the digestive tract discharge metabolic waste, and increase appetite to help digestion. It can also help purge and act as a diuretic. It can treat inappetence. Additionally, it can stop cough and dissolve phlegm.

Caution:
1) **Do not eat white radish with Wood Ear in the same meal. It might cause skin allergies.**
2) **Do not eat it with Apples in the same meal.**

The following are the benefits of consuming Mushrooms:
a) Mushrooms can reduce blood pressure, delay senility, and prevent constipation.
b) Mushrooms are anti-aging. The new technology proves that mushroom juice can make skin beautiful and antiaging.
c) Mushrooms also play a therapeutic role in diabetes, tuberculosis, infectious hepatitis, and neuritis and can be used for indigestion, constipation, and other diseases.

Caution:
Do not cook it; eat it with tomato and/or carrot in the same meal. It may reduce the nutrition of both foods, and you can lose the benefits of mushrooms.

Chapter 7

Aromatherapy and Massage Therapy

Your immune system becomes weak when you are tired and/or have body pain due to heavy bodywork or long hours. You must get a good rest to recover yourself.

I suggest you try Aromatherapy and combine it with massage therapy; use this on the painful parts of your body. Do it with your family members or friends, depending on your situation.

Research has shown that people can quickly recover and recharge by massaging with a pleasant, fragrant smell and/or soothing aromatherapy scent like in body oil. You may also listen to soft sounds of calming background music or ocean sounds while you rest for the night. A well-rested sleep could re-energize your body to work more efficiently for the new day.

The best amount of sleep is at least eight hours at night. Try to sleep before 10:00 pm, and you should wake up at 6 am. Based on medical research, data have shown that the human body is self-repairing the organs while they are asleep from 11:00 pm to 3:00 am.

With one exception, for example, when we travel to other countries with six to ten hours of time difference, we might find ourselves still in the sleeping schedule we are used to. Adjusting the physiological time difference will take three days to a week. This means that our body has the ability to adjust itself. Some people work night shifts; they develop their new routine sleeping cycles.

However, regular work and rest schedules are important and guarantee good health.

A thirty-minute to an hour nap after lunch is also an important way to re-energize your body for the afternoon.

SELF-MESSAGES ON HANDS FOR HEALING

According to a Traditional Chinese Medicine and Acupuncture Points study, messaging your hands daily may provide good maintenance for your five viscera and six entrails.

The Chinese Public Health Education (see the referenced pictures below) teaches us that many Acupuncture points on hands are related to human internal organs, such as the heart, spleen, liver, lungs, and kidneys.

When we feel some symptoms in the body, we can massage both hands entirely and focus on the specific area that reflects the corresponding body part to prevent a serious sickness from happening.

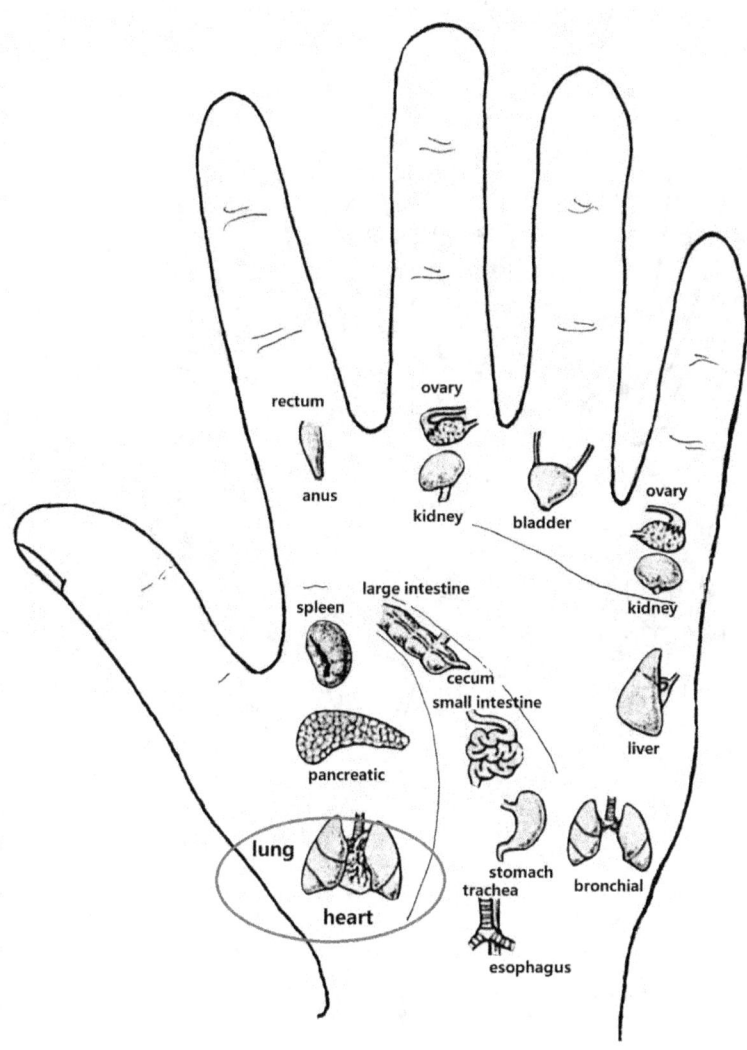

Left Hand

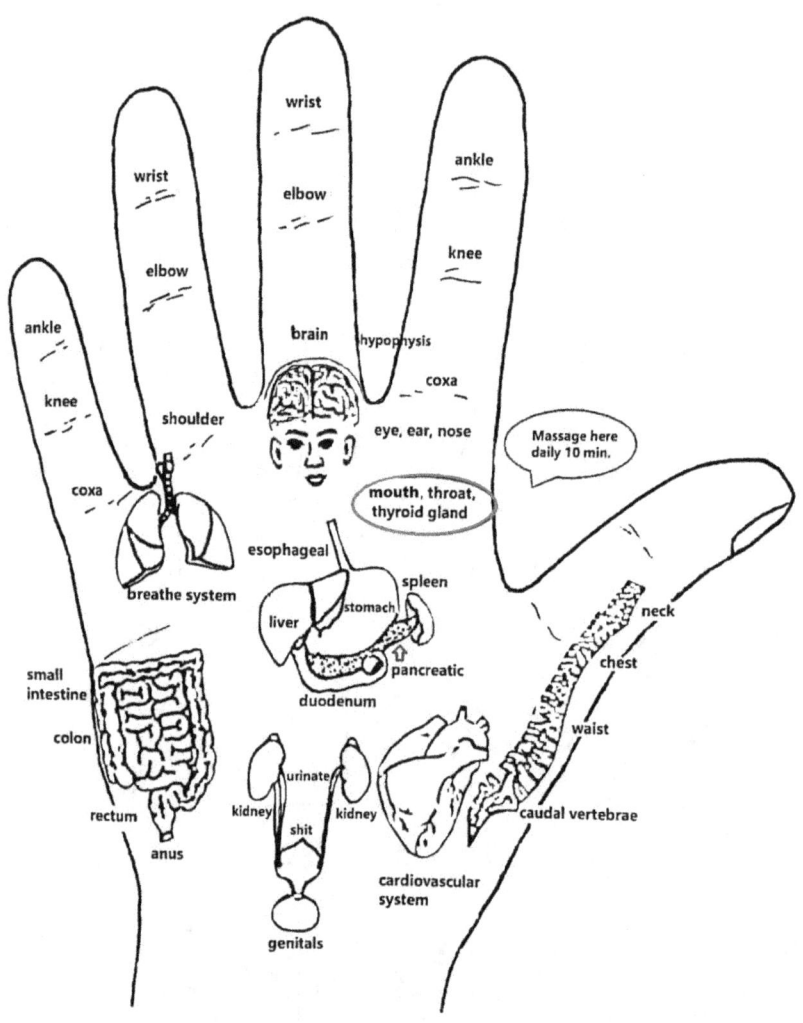

Right Hand

Reference 1 – Left-hand picture:
I used the red color circle in the place that indicates the lungs and heart on the left hand.

Reference 2 – Right-hand picture:
I used the red color circle in the place that indicates the mouth and throat on the right hand.

The COVID-19 Pandemic is attacking people's respiratory systems, as Hospitals reported sickness symptoms. It makes people sick; they cough and are unable to breathe well.

Message the two circled places on the hands above for ten minutes in the morning and ten minutes before bedtime. This will help improve the functioning of the lungs and throat. Therefore, you can stay healthy during/after the COVID-19 Pandemic.

Chapter 8

Daily Exercise

People do many types of exercises to stay healthy. The most common are yoga, Tai Chi, and School health exercises. Yoga is a good discipline for learning to relax. Yoga is usually combined with meditation to stay mentally calm. Tai chi is an ancient form of self-defense. It focuses on internal Qi that circulates inside the body.

From elementary to high school, we do health exercises and eye exercises at 10:00 am, which is between the four classes in the morning.

No matter what kind of exercise you do, do one daily to stay healthy.

Some people like to do yoga before sleeping at night. Occasionally, I exercise at night before sleeping. If I miss my morning exercise due to a busy schedule, I always make it up with some other work, like sweeping the floor, mopping the floor, cleaning the kitchen, etc.

There are three basic daily physical exercises for staying healthier:
1. Get up in the morning and do the body stretchy exercise you usually do.
2. Walk at least thirty minutes per day.
3. There are many Acupuncture points on our two hands that can treat shoulder, neck, and other types of body pain. Doing some self-massage on your hands' Acupuncture points will help you stay healthy.

Exercise is good for the brain. Exercise can be done in two forms: (1) Exercising your body through work, such as yard work, sweeping and mopping the floor, etc., and (2) Exercising at a Fitness Center.

When your body moves, your heart actively pumps blood through your blood vessels, keeping your body active and healthy.

This exercise strategy is especially important for people who work in the Office and/or at Home. Exercising daily can help you stay healthy and get work done more efficiently.

Chapter 9

Treat Dark Spots and Skin Tags

The most common skin issues are dark spots, skin tags, freckles, age spots, moles, and warts. Everyone wants clean and beautiful skin, especially on the face. The good news is that technology is developing, and many new and improved products are available in the market to help people resolve those skin issues.

Freckle are caused by long time exposures under Sunlight for teenagers. For older adult, we see some age spot on hands, arms, and face. I have tested many products. I suggest using PFMC Fade Cream to treat freckle and age spot. If the brown spot cannot be removed by the Fade Cream, try the Skin Tag Remover product. The Skin Tag Remover can help remove the mole and wart as well. See product pictures below for your references.

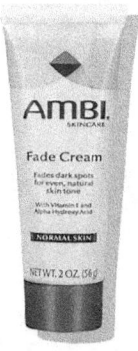 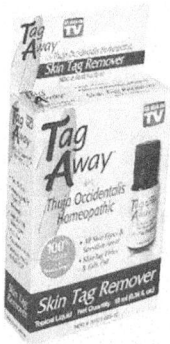

Pimple are caused by the hair follicle being blocked by the oil on the skin's surface. Acne is caused by clogged follicles. It shows some oil and dead skin cells leading to whiteheads and blackheads. Acne and Pimple come and go as we keep up the treatment on the face. It associated with the meals, especially when you eat a big meal with fried chicken or any food that has a lot of fatty parts on it.

These are some solutions:

(a) Eat less fatty meat and more vegetables; this will improve the Acne skin.
(b) Drinking Green Tea will help remove some extra fat from the meals that we have eaten.
(c) Use the skin of fruit (the inside part) to message the face to remove the extra oil that accumulated during the day from exploring to outdoor activities. Use fruits such as, Banana, orange, Apple, and watermelon.

Use banana skin to treat Wart on the face. Use the inside part of banana skins to massage the face, especially the Wart. Slowly you might see an improvement and get cleaner skin on your face.

Use homemade Skin Fade method to remove the dark color spots. You will need the following materials:

a) One egg (use the white part only and take the yoke out)
b) One inch of Toothpaste (whitening formula)
c) Two spoonful of Vinegar
d) Two spoonful of milk

Mix them well.

Before you take a shower before going to bed, rub the Home-Made Fade Solution (liquid) on your face, neck and arms skin and gently massage your skin for about ten to twenty minutes, then wash it out with warm water.

Putting a small amount of lotion on your skin before sleeping.

You will see a significant result of clearer and lighter skin on your face after you continuously use it for one month.

Chapter 10

Healing Dry Skin and Skin Maintenance

Dry skin can be healed by putting Petroleum jelly on the skin every day after washing and/or showering.

If the skin on your whole body is feeling dry and itch and if you see some white skin flaking or creasing due to dryness, you can use moisture soap to wash your body. Then apply some Baby Oil or Coconut Body Oil on your skin and message it for about ten minutes without rinsing it out.

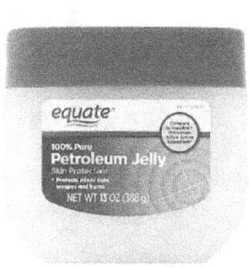 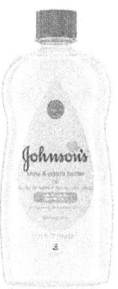 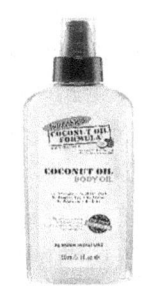

Petroleum Jelly   Baby Oil   Coconut Oil for Body

Continue the Petroleum Jelly and Body Oil treatment for ten days. You will see a significantly improved result on your skin.

HOMEMADE MOISTURIZE WATER FOR STOPPING ITCH AND DRY SKIN IN WINTER

During the Winter time, when you feel itch on skin, you spray some of your own home-made Body Moisturize Water on your body skin to heal the dry skin and stop the itch.

You will need the following materials:

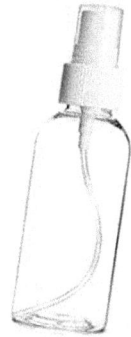 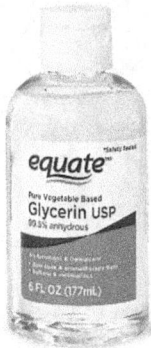 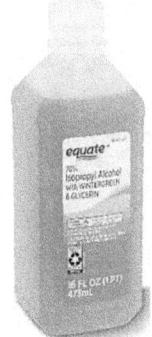

Spray bottle   Glycerin   Isopropyl Alcohol

1. Grab an empty spray bottle.
2. Add purified drinking water into the bottle (75 percent of the bottle).
3. Add glycerin into the spray bottle (20 percent of the bottle).
4. Add 15 ml of 70% Alcohol with Winter Green.

Mix them well, and it will be ready to use.

OVERALL SKIN MAINTENANCE METHODS

Treat the Mosquito bit during the Summertime. Currently the most powerful product for healing the Mosquitoes bit is the Cutter® Insect Repellent. I suggest you have at least two bottles handy for your family's need during the Summer each year.

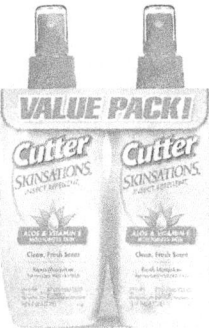

When you have skin rash due to Allergies or Poisonous Plants and are scratching on your legs or hands, use the over-the-counter medicine Cortizone 10.

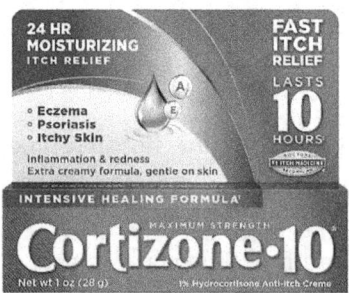

To avoid Sun Burn, putting some Sun Block Lotion on the face, neck, arms, and legs where your skin is exposure to the Sunlight. During the Summertime, we often experience a Sunburn situation when we go to beach to swim or hike in the mountains for outdoor activities.

Chapter 11

Facial Massage for a Younger-Looking Face

Getting a facial massage is a great method to keep skin tight and look young and beautiful for a longer time. *Use Facial Oil to massage your face.*

For references, I selected a few of the facial oil product based on the function that we need it to have, and the prices are below $15.00 per bottle.

Caution: Avoid getting the oil into your eyes. In case you have a little oil in your eye by accident, rinse your eye with plenty of cold water for about five minutes. Putting a drop of the Opcon-A® Eye Allergy Relief eye drops into each eye can help avoid eye irritation along with redness, itch, and allergy symptoms.

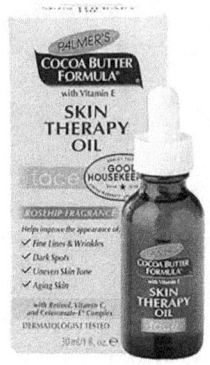
Skin Therapy Oil

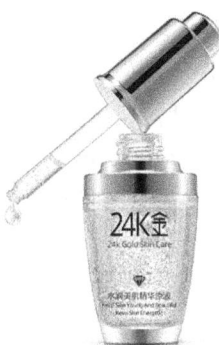
Anti-aging face oil

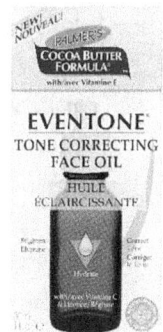
Tone Correcting Face Oil

Here are different methods you can use for your facial massage:

1. To reduce eye bags, use the third finger (also called ring finger) to put a drop of face oil on each of eye bag and massage it, going from the eye's inner corner to the outside corner. Then move your fingers up a little to your eyelid and gently massage your eyelid skin from the outer corner to inner corner of the eye. Massage your eye by gently moving your third fingers around your eye. Softly move your finger around the eye for about ten times.
2. Massage the forehead with both hands from the center of forehead to each side. Do it ten times.
3. Use your two thumbs to massage the area behind each ear. Putting a little bit of pressure on it and move up and down ten to twenty times.
4. Massage your cheeks with both hands. Starting from the jaw and chin, move slowly up to the top of your head. Do it ten times.
5. Use your index and middle fingers together to massage the point beside the nose. Move your two fingers at the same point in circle for ten times. Put a little pressure on the points to prevent Rhinitis Coryza (also called Nasitis).
6. For students, use your index finger and the tumble to hold the Glabella and eye socket and massage it. It can help you relax your eye after a long hour of reading.
7. For girls, please avoid reading on the computer for long time while you have your monthly menstruation because the loss of blood might weaken your eyesight if you continuously use your eyes for more than two hours. Take a break and relax your eyes for ten minutes before going back to your desk to read again if you have to get some reading and writing work done.
8. Message your ears for a few minutes each day. Press your ears with your hands then release. You will feel the air being pumped out from the ears. It can help loosen some earwax.

9. Use both your middle fingers to massage the sides of your nose. From the sides of your nostrils, move up to the top of forehead then move down to the sides of nostrils again. Move slowly with a little pressure from the middle fingers. Do this ten times.
10. Use your ten fingers to comb your hair thoroughly from the forehead to the back end at neck. Do it ten times.
11. Massage your jaw, starting from the behind the ears to the jaw and chin. Use your right hand to massage the left side from behind the ear to the chin. Use your left hand to massage the right side from behind the ear to the chin.

Chapter 12

Eczema Treatment

Why do people have Eczema? Eczema is mainly caused by genetic factors and environmental factors. Genetic factor are from inside the body; There is a protein has a genetic mutation. It can be passed from parents to children. The external factors that trigger eczema include moist/humid/damp environments; this can damage the skin.

a) If the eczema is caused by living in a humid environment, you need to improve your living environment. For example, some people live in the basement rooms. It might cause them to have eczema, especially when their parent has a history of eczema. Genetically they can get the eczema problem really fast when exposed to the moist/humid/damp environment.

b) If the eczema is caused by a lack of exercise and physical work/activity, you need to do some more exercise to help your body sweat out the extra water under your skin. Do remember to drink some water slowly during the physical work and sweat times to avoid dehydration.

c) If the eczema is caused by your sleeping schedule (for example, sleeping too late and not getting up in the morning on time), you need to change your daily schedule to have a healthy sleeping habit.

d) Do not overeat. Overeat will cause the problem of subcutaneous fat accumulation. When there is too much fat under the skin, it could block your sweat from coming out, which can cause metabolic disorders.

Here are some treatment methods for eczema:

a) Drink Green Tea in the morning after breakfast. Tea could help people's urine system to urinating the excess water out.

  Note: Do not drink tea after 4:00 pm because the tea contains some theophylline which can make people awake for a few hours. Most people have the sleeping schedule at 9:00 pm or 10:00 pm. We want to sleep well after the whole day's work and/or study without anything that might disturb our sleep.

b) Life need water. We should have eight cups of water each day to maintain a good, healthy body. And the body will urinate the extra body waste out.

c) Eat three meals per day and on time with your daily schedule. Do not wait until you are hungry to eat. Eat meals at the standard hours. For example, Breakfast is from 6:00 am to 7:00 am. Lunch hour is from noon to 1:00 pm. Dinnertime is during 6:00 pm to 8:00 pm.

d) Use Food Medicine. Some Vegetables and fruit are particularly good for digestion and can help the urinary system remove excess moisture, for example, Radish, Red beans, Mung Beans, peanuts, potatoes, carrots, ginger, millet, yellow corn, lotus seeds, pumpkin, yam and so on.

e) Some Fruits are good for the functioning of the spleen by removing the extra moisture in body, for example, watermelon, orange, mango, papaya, pineapple, yellow peach, sweet pear, banana, etc.

f) In addition, often stimulating and patting some associated acupuncture points are also can remove moisture.

Chapter 13

Hair Loss Treatment

The hair loss is caused by heredity, hormonal changes, or medical conditions and is also a normal part of aging. Excessive hair loss from your scalp can make you bald.

The most common reason is age. Have confidence to have a beautiful hair again. There are many products available in the market now for growing your hair back.

I introduce to you the most economic and affordable (less than $10.00 per bottle) product: *Regrow 7 Day Ginger Germinal Hair Growth Serum Loss Treatment Oil (30ml)*. See picture below.

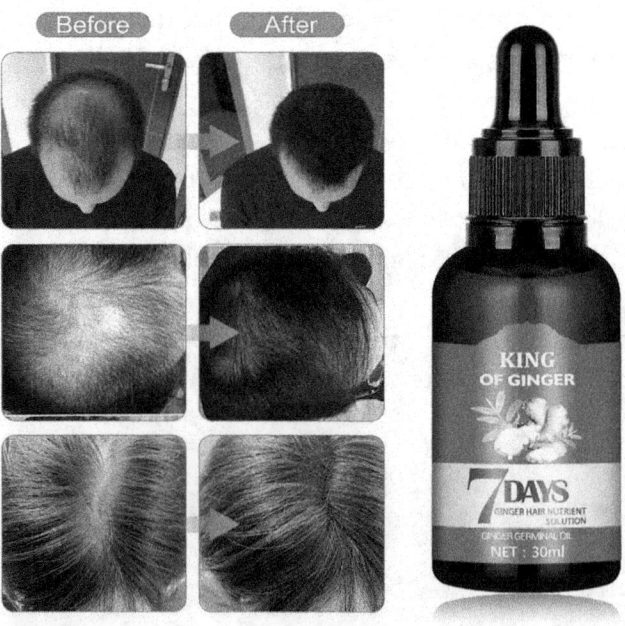

There are a few methods to maintain beautiful hair. There is also a method that we can use in our personal cleanliness to avoid the hair loss.

For oily hair, we use a spoonful of Baking Soda add to warm water and wash your hair with it once per week to remove the extra oil buildup from the scalp.

For dry hair, massage some olive oil or coconut oil into the ends of your hair, where the split ends are.

Chapter 14

Red Eye & Itchy Eye Treatment

Pink eye is a common disease that it is a type of bacterial infection. The symptoms are red and swollen eyes, itchy, painful, and/or dry eyes, pricking eye, excess tears, fear of light, more discharge than usual, etc. Giving timely treatment will help you recover soon.

It could be caused by pollen, dust, or something floating in the work environment that lends in your eyes. People always feel like wanting to rub with their hands when something irritate the eyes. Rubbing with unclean hands might make the eyelids swell and cause eye inflammation.

Here are some quick methods to resolve the situations:
a) Water rinse treatment: Rinse your eyes with clean water for a few seconds. Pad dry with a clean towel or paper towel with the eyes closed to avoid anything touching the eyes directly.
b) Use Moisturizes Eye Drops or a Redness Relieve Eye Drop solution to clear the eyes. They are available at Walmart Stores for $0.97 per 0.5 FL OZ bottle. Putting a few drops of the Moisturizes Eye Drop solution to clean out any particles out from the eyes. This works if you use it immediately after feeling the irritation.

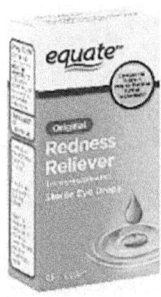

c) Use Eye Allergy Relief solution to treat pink eye. When you have a large amount of sticky yellowish or white substance at the cornea, it can lead to blurred vision. Clean it out with a clean towel and warm water. Use the Eye Allergy Relief eye drops immediately.

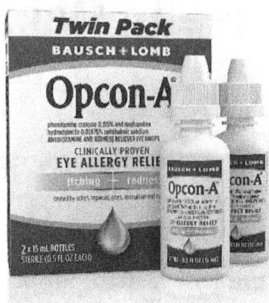

This is the most efficient Eye Allergy Relief solution that is available without a prescription.

Have a good, healthy reading habit. Sit at Desk and keep at least one foot between your eyes and your reading target (such as computer screens and books).

Chapter 15

Hearing Health Maintenance

Deafness can be inherited, or it can be acquired due to inflammation or nerve disease. If you experience significant hearing loss, you must go to see doctors in the hospital for treatment to avoid serious damage to your hearing and permanent hearing impairment.

How do we maintain good hearing Health?

a) Protect your ears in daily life. Avoid infection caused by dirty water entering in the ears when you wash face and hair. Use a clean Cotton Swab gently wipe the ear if you feel some water get into it.
b) Do not stay in a noisy environment often. Hearing loss could be caused by loud music and loud noises. If you work in construction industry or manufacturing industry, some machines make loud noises that you must use earplug that can help reduce the sound volumes of noise to protect your ears.
c) Some people like to use headset. You make sure the volumes is not too loud for your ears. You need to take breaks from the headset every two to three hours.
d) To remove earwax, use a Cotton Swab and wet the tip into Hydrogen Peroxide Tropical Solution (First Aid Antiseptic). Gently clean the earwax out. Usually, the earwax comes out itself without cleaning. You only need to clean it when you feel a little itch or irritation inside the ear.

e) Massage your ears daily for five minutes. If you do health exercise daily, it should be included in the exercise already.

Step 1: Use your hands to rub both of ears up and down for ten times.

Step 2: Use your index fingers to gently insert to both ears and move around up and down two times and quickly take fingers out as you are taking a small piece of dried earwax out.

Step 3: Repeat step 2 twice.

Chapter 16

Car Sickness Treatment

MODERN MEDICINE METHOD

Take a motion sickness pill before traveling by car or by airplane. For people who are wary of the side effects of medicine, the Herb Method might be the best option for car sickness treatment.

HERB METHOD

Put a slice of Ginger on your belly bottom by taping it with a bandage. When you feel carsick, use your hand to push down on your belly bottom where the Ginger is sitting, then take deep breaths slowly; breathe in through your nose and breathe out through your mouth until the symptom reduced to the level you can handle.

HAND MASSAGE METHOD

Use your thumb and index finger to hold the point (also called Hegu point in traditional Chinese Medical Practice) between the opposite thumb and index finger. Use your right hand to massage your left hand. Then use your left hand to massage your right hand. Do it whenever you need it to stop feeling like throwing up from car sickness.

FRESH AIR METHOD

Sit at the front seat and near the window if you have car sickness situation. If you feel dizzy, you open the window to have some fresh air to blow onto your face. The fresh air method could stop the car sickness and dizziness and avoid vomiting.

Chapter 17

Slam Your Fat Belly

METHOD 1: EXERCISE

Tighten your belly muscle with a simple exercise.

a) Stand straight and hold the chair's high back. Look forward far and keep your neck straight.
b) Move your RIGHT leg backward as far as you can until you feel your belly muscle is tightening from the leg movement. Repeat this ten times.
c) Move your LEFT leg backward as far as you can until you feel your belly muscle tightening from the leg movement. Repeat this ten times.

Do this exercise whenever you have a chance at Office and at home.

METHOD 2: GINGER TREATMENT ON BELLY BOTTOM

In the market, there are so many kinds of Weight Loss products now. You can select a few of them to try based on your personal situation.

The most common fat person is growing extra fat everywhere on the body. We usually consider it caused by overeating, or the habit of consuming too much fatty meat in each meal.

In this book, I share a traditional herbal method to slam the Fat Belly caused by heavy moisture (called shiqi in Chinese Medicine).

Some people get a big fat belly by drinking too much Beer. Some people get a big fat belly by eating a big meal with a lot of meat late night from 10:00 pm to 12:00 am before sleeping.

What is shiqi? *Shiqi* is a condition where there is water retention/"dampness" in the body from excessive accumulation of moisture and not having it discharged in time. Years of fatigue can lead to decreased metabolism and bad lifestyle habits. When the weather is hot, the body becomes hot and damp, and when the weather is cold, it becomes cold and damp. Everyone's situation is different, so you need a targeted therapy guided by Chinese Herb Doctors.

To completely remove the extra moisture in the body, people must start by treating the spleen and stomach. Sometimes, it is difficult to dispel using common methods. In that case, you need to do targeted body recovery.

First, we need to know what kind of situation caused the belly to be bigger than other parts of our body. For example, if the belly is growing so much fat that it's bigger than the arms and legs, it might be a physical sickness -- shiqi.

Shiqi could also cause eczema or a fungal infection on your hands or feet. When it is on the feet, it called Athlete's Food. I will write these two common skin issues' treatment methods in a separate chapter.

Secondly, I suggest you begin adjusting your lifestyle. Have a balanced work and rest schedule to rest well each night. Do not stay up late. Get up at 5:00 am or 6:00 am and sleep before 10:00 pm. Do some exercises each day to give the body a good restorative environment. Take a nap after lunch if needed.

Eat some food that is good for spleen and for clearing up the dampness (with respect to diet). It is particularly important to avoid eating a big meal with a lot of meat after 10:00 pm and right before sleeping at night.

Thirdly, I will introduce to you a good method that use a natural plant – Ginger -- to ensure safety and no harm on the body. This method has been proven to help people who have had many years of heat and dampness coexisting accompanied by various concurrent symptoms like insomnia, bad breath, acne, bad stomach, car sickness, etc.

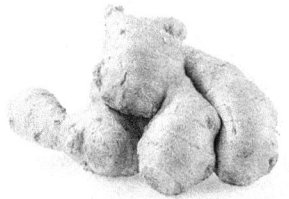

Ginger

1. Cut one piece of fresh Ginger into small pieces.
2. Dip a cotton swab in a little 70% Isopropyl Alcohol to gently clean your belly button.
3. Put some small Ginger pieces on the belly button.
4. Add one drop of Vinegar on top of the Ginger pieces at the belly button.
5. Tape the Ginger to the belly button with a large bandage.

   Optional: For people who want to lose more fat on the belly, you can use a new and clean plastic bag (large 33 gal. size) around your belly (with the fresh Ginger pieces at the belly button) tightly before sleeping. It might make some sweat come out from the belly. Clean it out with warm water when you wake up in the morning.

   Continue doing it for a month. You will feel that the Ginger method restored the metabolism of your spleen and stomach so that moisture will not relapse. The symptoms of insomnia, halitosis, acne, obesity, sweating, chills, etc. will completely disappear or at least visibly improve, depending on each person's body condition.

METHOD 3: GINGER, BLACK PEPPER, AND DRIED RED DATES JUICE

Use ginger, black pepper, and red dates as food medicine to help discharge the extra wet and fatty from eating fatty foods that caused the fat belly.

Materials needed: six pieces of dates, 3g of black pepper, a large piece of ginger

Preparation: Cut the ginger into small pieces. Clean the dates. See picture below.

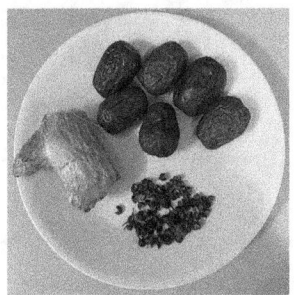 →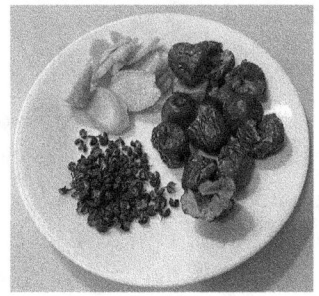

Dates, pepper, ginger   Cut ginger, remove cores

Use a pot to cook the ginger and dried red dates with a full bowel of water. When the water is boiled, turn the stove on low/medium heat to cook the ginger and dates together for fifteen minutes. You can add some brown sugar for better taste. Eat the dates and ginger. Drink the juice. Take this food medicine daily for three days, when you feel that you need it. Ginger can make you feel warm.

Note: Do not add sugar for diabetes patient.

METHOD 4: APPLE AND DATES JUICE

Use apple and red dates as food medicine to help discharge the extra wet and fatty from eating fatty foods that caused the fat belly.

Materials needed: six pieces of dates, an apple, black pepper is optional to add or not add. Apple can slam the fat belly.

Preparation: Cut the apple into small pieces. Clean the dates.

See picture below.

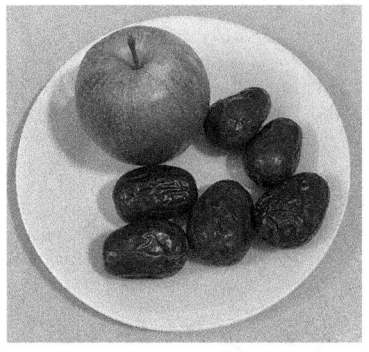
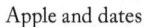
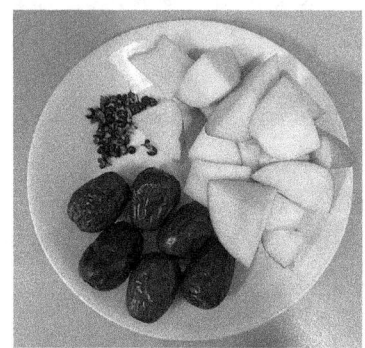

Apple and dates   Cut apple to small pieces

Use a pot to cook the apple pieces and dried red dates with a full bowel of water. When the water is boiled, turn the stove on low/medium heat to cook the apple and dates together for fifteen minutes. You can add some brown sugar for better taste. Eat the dates and apple. Drink the juice. Take this food medicine daily for three days when you feel that you need it.

Chapter 18

Body Cramp Treatment

When we say "body cramp," we usually mean leg cramp, arm cramp, and hand cramp. The main cause of cramps is a lack of movement for a long time; there is a sudden increase momentum, causing strain on the muscle (e.g., the gastrocnemius muscle on the leg) or fascia inflammation. There is abnormal discharge, and the phenomenon of muscle twitching appears.

Personally, I have experienced leg cramps many times myself in my teenage years when I swam two to three extra hours. Sometimes my leg or foot cramped in that situation. Here is the urgent care I learned from my parents: Do not try to bend the leg or foot. Do not touch it. Let your body relax. After five to ten minutes of relaxing, my leg and foot started becoming soft and could move freely again, which meant it was back to normal. However, it was time for me to stop the swimming activity.

These are some treatment recommendations for cramps:
a) Maintain adequate rest and reduce leg weight-bearing activities when the body cramp happens.
b) To avoid cramps, exercise your body daily to build up strong muscles on your arms and legs. Gradually increase exercise or the amount of activity under your coach's advice. Do a good amount of warm-up activities before a big event.
c) Apply hot compress. Massage and physiotherapy can also be used to promote blood circulation.
d) Take an appropriate amount of calcium supplements.

If the pain persists for a long time, you need to go to the orthopedic department of the hospital for further examination and treatment.

Chapter 19

Treatment for Athlete's Foot

Before sleeping at night, soak your feet into warm salt water for ten minutes. Dry your feet with a clean dry towel, then sprinkle some baby powder to treat the wetness between the toes. Do it daily.

Athlete's foot is a skin problem on the feet and can be transferred through shoes. For example, if you wear someone else's shoe and they have athlete's foot, you could get the same problem from the dirty shoe. Do not wear your friend's shoe when you know they have athlete's foot.

You need to treat the stinky shoe. Athlete's foot can make their shoes stinky. Mash two mothballs into powder then sprinkle the powder into each shoe. Mothballs not only kill clothes moths and their eggs and larvae but also remove the stinky smell in the shoe.

Chapter 20

Sauna Bath: Benefits and Caution

A sauna is also known as a Finnish bath because the sauna originated in Finland and dates back to more than two thousand years. It is a process of physical therapy using steam in an enclosed room. The temperature in the sauna can reach up to and above 60 °C. It uses steam produced from pouring cold water on hot rocks to wash the body. This makes the blood vessels repeatedly dilate and contract and can enhance Hemal elasticity. It can, therefore, prevent Hemal sclerosis.

Saunas can speed up blood circulation to make the muscles of each part of the body completely relax. It can eliminate fatigue, restore physical strength, and feeling mentally energized. Plus, using the sauna has certain effects on rheumatism, arthritis, back pain, asthma, bronchitis, neurasthenia, etc. In addition, the traditional sauna has an inherent health care effect. It is a kind of enjoyment and leisure activity and is a treat for the overworked body of working-class people.

High-temperature environments have an effect on our skin-deep internal heat; there is a systemic capillary expansion, causing the body to sweat much more than when doing ordinary activities at other times. This carefree sweating is conducive to the discharge of various garbage and toxins inside the body and is also conducive to the elimination of diseases such as skin problems.

In the wintertime at the very cold northern part of the Earth, temperatures could go down to -10 °C. It is understandable that people created the sauna to survive the cold weather.

I remember that some students said, "The cold is getting into my bones in the late winter night," while they came back home from studying and research activities at the university. This was when I was living in the northern part of the United States. We shared a method of taking *hot* baths to remove the cold from body.

I had enjoyed ice fishing in the wintertime when the lake was frozen over. We drilled a hole about twelve inches wide and caught many fish there. Sometimes my body felt so cold during the fishing activity that we had to go back home early. I found a good way to recover from the cold, and that uses the concept of the sauna.

First, I rinse my body with warm water for a few minutes while I clean the bathtub.

Secondly, I soak my body in *hot* water that is about 40 °C—a temperature my body can tolerate—for about thirty minutes and finish the bath with soap.

Finally, I then rinse my body with warm water for a minute before coming out.

This is an easy way to treat *cold* away from the body at home when there is no sauna facility near your residential community.

Caution: Medical experts have warned that frequent visits to the sauna could be a major cause of male infertility due to the high temperature.

For senior people who have heart diseases, they must consult with a doctor before doing sauna.

Chapter 21

Diabetes Care and Sugar Control in Meals

Based on medical research and study, diabetes is related to genetics and environmental factors. It should be noted that the genetic background only gives individuals a certain degree of susceptibility to diabetes; it's not enough to cause the disease.

Diabetes is generally caused by the overall effect of multiple genetic abnormalities under the action of environmental factors—eating habits, lifestyles, lack of daily exercising, etc.

Eating sugar will not lead to diabetes, but if you eat too much sugar for a long time, it will increase the burden of the pancreas and induce obesity, which is a risk factor that leads to the occurrence of diabetes.

To avoid the threat of diabetes, we must eat a balanced diet and maintain a healthy lifestyle.

In healthy individuals, if the pancreas is functioning properly, when food enters the body, sugar is broken down into glucose. Glucose then passes into the bloodstream and becomes blood sugar. Elevated blood sugar levels stimulate the beta cells in the pancreas to secrete insulin, which lowers blood sugar levels and keeps glucose levels in the blood within the normal range.

Reference ranges: Normal fasting condition blood glucose is 3.9–6.1 mmol/L. Normal postprandial blood glucose is 7.8–11.1 mmol/L

Whether the blood glucose is high or not depends on whether the blood glucose is measured on an empty stomach or after a meal. The target blood glucose levels for diabetic patients needs to be based on the patient's condition, complications caused by diabetes, as well as their age so as to establish the most suitable target level of blood glucose.

For some people who have lived with bad lifestyle habits for years (either one of these or a combination of the following: alcohol, obesity, overeating, loving sweets, etc.), these habits will increase the burden on the body's regulation of blood sugar.

Here are things you can do to manage the blood sugar and keep it within the normal ranges:

a) Eat fruits that contain less sugar such as apple, orange, pear, etc. Eat a variety of fruit each week.
b) Use less oil in dishes. Cook healthier food by steaming instead of using oil to fry.
c) Fish and shrimp contain less fat than pork and beef. Therefore, eating less pork and beef is good for health.

What kind of food is good for managing diabetes? Green leafy vegetables, corn, buckwheat, wheat bran, soybeans, black beans, bitter melon, etc. have low glycemic effect and rich dietary fiber; these have certain effects on blood glucose control.

Chapter 22

Balance Body Energy for Mind Wellness

Physical wellness is a combination of living well with the daily schedule of study (for students), working well (for adults), eating three meals (breakfast, lunch, and dinner) on time, and resting well at night.

Physical wellness brings family happiness. Sometimes, we might encounter a stressful situation that we can't handle. All we need to do is Trust God. If you cannot resolve it, God can. Just let God take care of it for you. Then we go to do something that we can help ourselves.

Seventeen years ago, my right hand was broken due to a fall on the ground at Skating Land. I thought positively that my hand was broken, so my daughter's hands and legs were saved. Because she asked me to take her to play at the four-wheel shoe Skating Land every weekend.

I could not care for my two children, aged ten and six, at home anymore. So, I prayed to God, asking him to take care of them for me and to make them useful and helpful. God listened and helped. Now, they both have completed their college education and are working.

According to a recent study by researchers, religious practice may be beneficial to physical and mental health. Researchers at Duke University Medical Center in the United States conducted a series of studies to explore the relationship between religion and human health. The result is promisingly good and healthy.

There are what the Bible teaches:

a) God cares about you personally. – Peter 5:7
b) God's personal name is Jehovah. – Psalm 83:18
c) Jehovah invites you to draw close to him. – James 4:8
d) Jehovah is loving, kind, and merciful. – Exodus 34:6; 1 John 4:8, 16

The three major religions in the world are Buddhism, Christianity, and Islam. They all believe in God.

God is real. God wants the Earth filled with healthy people. Please see the below-referenced picture from the book <<What Does the Bible Really Teach?>>.

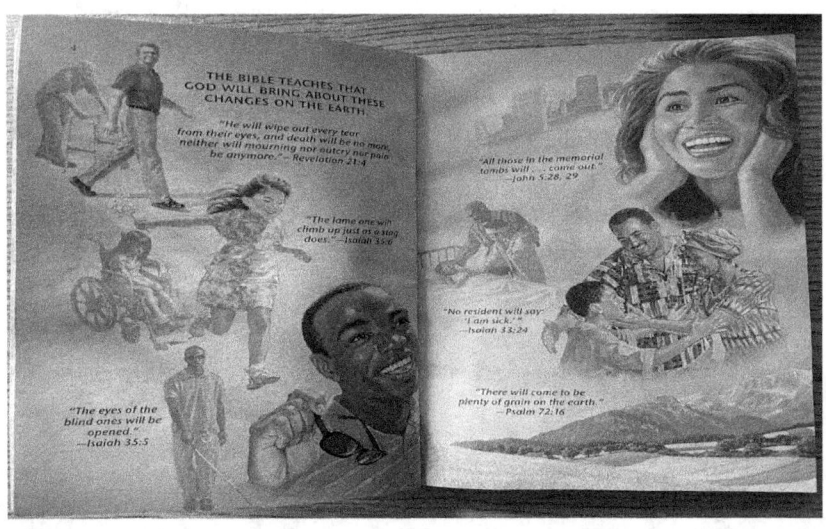

I trust God. I work for God. I work on projects that contribute toward fulfilling God's plan to help people become healthier and happier.

I have heard people say, "The medical bill is so high, we can't afford it," or "We may go bankrupt for the medical expenses." Some people say, "We have to take painkiller drugs every day because my body is hurting." "I am so tired that I have to drink 3 cups of Coffee to keep me awake." "I am so tired, and I have to smoke to reenergize again." It all means that they need a good rest to recover their bodies.

Some drugs can temporarily energize people, but after a certain time, it makes people even more tired. It makes people attached to the drug again and again.

Some people increase their dosages for painkiller drugs. They eventually die from overdosage.

Some people increase their dosages of energizing drugs, so that their health becomes damaged. The drug can cause people depression, based on medical research and studies.

No medicine can make people strong. Medicine is for healing some sickness. All medicines have some side effects, so we must take them according to a doctor's guidelines.

People become stronger and stronger through work. Athletes build up their muscles and skills through years of training day by day!

This book, <<How to Stay Healthy>>, provides some information on food function, Herbs, and methods for using them. Some food medicine methods were used in ancient times to treat some sicknesses and symptoms. They are affordable, low-cost, and doable at home to help people become Healthier & Happier!

Balance your body's energy through healthy lifestyle habits and scheduling time for Mind Wellness.

Healthy lifestyle habits include the four major parts:

a) Eat well.

Have some fruit and vegetables daily. Drink enough water to avoid dehydration.

b) Work well.

Many people get enough body exercise at their jobs. Office workers need to schedule physical exercise for about twenty to thirty minutes daily in the morning or evening to stay in good body shape.

Athletes have strong and healthy bodies built up with daily exercises and years of effort.

c) Sleep well.

Our body gets re-energized during sleep time. Medical research shows that the cells in our body adjust and repair themselves to fit our body's needs. Have eight hours of sleep each day and go to bed by 10:00 pm.

d) Meditation well.

If you don't know yoga or other methods, just closing your eyes and listening to music can be meditation. Your mind becomes calm and clear when you do the twenty minutes meditation daily.

Chapter 23

Goal Setting for Your Career Success

A healthy body starts with a healthy mind. Goal-setting is great for adults and students. Write down the weekly and monthly goals you want to accomplish in your career. Study while following a daily exercise plan and schedule to maintain a healthy body. From this, you have a good, healthy body to accomplish your goals every day.

Setting a long-term goal for the year is also important for achieving your career goal. Once you have the year's goal set, you will be able to look at it from your current point of view to see how much work you need to do to accomplish the goal. This way, you can schedule and manage your daily life more efficiently.

In life, we get some unexpected situations that might delay our schedule to reach the goal. We must forgive ourselves as we often forgive others. My advice is to treat yourself to a nice meal. Rest well to recover your body's energy first to overcome the unexpected situation. Plan a day or a week to catch up with some workload so you will feel better again.

Life has ups and downs. Stay modest in the ups and keep self-respect in the downs. Trust God and know that everything will come to pass. The important thing is to learn from it. Do better soon.

In the career competition, other people cannot fail you. Only you can fail yourself. Make sure your goal-setting is in good faith. Get back to work again after recharging your body's energy through resting, massaging, and love. Love is the cure and answer for many problems in one's personal life. Love has healing power! When our hearts are filled with love, there is no space for problems.

A career success often takes more time than just working from 9:00 a.m. to 5:00 p.m. Loving what you do and doing what you love is the key to success in your career. Every professional person can tell you that they have put much of their spare time into working to build their career. That is why people say, "Making your habit into your business is the best way to success." It's because your habit is what you love to do, even you don't get paid for doing it. It means you work for yourself to make yourself happy instead of working for others for money.

Telling yourself to "just do it" is a powerful way to accomplish your career goal. You forget the hours and labor. All your focus is on getting it done. In fact, you will be rewarded for the long term in life after you accomplish your career goal.

A car needs a good maintenance to keep running well. The human body also needs good care and health maintenance to stay away from sickness. Whenever you feel a little symptom or that you do not feel well, try some of those methods in this handbook to stay healthy and strong.

www.ingramcontent.com/pod-product-compliance
Lightning Source LLC
LaVergne TN
LVHW011739060526
838200LV00051B/3246